Air Fryer Toaster Oven Cookbook

Quick, Easy and Delicious Air Fryer
Oven Recipes for Healthy Meals

Introduction

An air fryer oven is an easy way to cook delicious healthy meals. If you cook your food in oil, it may affect your health but in an air fryer food cooks oil free. An air fryer oven machine uses rapid hot air to circulate around the food. This allows to cook many dishes with meat, vegetables, poultry, fruit, fish and a wide variety of desserts.

It is a safer method of cooking and you get the ability to set and leave food to cook most models that have a digital timer. Air fryer cooks can bake, grill, roast and fry providing more options.

Although, air fryer toaster oven cooking seems new, professional chefs have been using it for decades in commercial kitchens for its speed and cooking and browning features. Today these ovens are widely available to home cooks at affordable prices.

There are millions of air fryer toaster ovens in private homes today, but people have had to figure out on their own how to adapt their favorite recipes, with varying°of success. This book is here to help!

Air fryers work by distributing incredibly hot air around the food and don't require oil or fat. You can add a tiny amount to boost taste if you want, however, this generally just a teaspoon full. Which means they are best for anyone and everyone who enjoys yummy healthier food.

They're especially helpful for people who are counting the calories. Dieting may be challenging and usually rules out any fried foods, just from the nature in which they're cooked. Air fryers aren't only for chips! Any sort of food, from chicken bits to pineapple rings could be cooked this manner. The only limiting factor is your own imagination.

The air filter removes the need for a nasty skillet at the house. They're practical and simple to wash and make a fantastic addition to any kitchen.

The fryer functions by directing a heated flow of air over and about the food that's placed in a basket. The basket is stored in a drawer that slots to the front part of the appliance - hence no longer lowering of meals to hot oil. You choose the cooking temperature using a thermostat which is simple, and also the time using a detachable timer. The fryer turns itself off in the end. To cook over 1 food item, simply use the basket divider. This underlines the flexibility of this machine. It's really just like a convection oven setup using a basket to let it manage foods that would usually go in the deep fryer.

It occupies bit more room than a normal sized food processor, also seems impressive and futuristic. Since all the components that contact the meals are all dishwasher-safe, it's simple to stay clean.

It comes using a fast start guide to get you moving, in addition to a detailed recipe book with 250 distinct recipes that you try, you will be amazed by the assortment of unexpected foods which you may cook at the air fryer...

Chapter 1: Understand an air fryer toaster oven

These days, most new full-size and built-in air fryer toaster ovens come with an air fryer function, but here's a sad truth: Most people don't use the air fryer function on their ovens. Why? Because they don't know how to.

Air circulation doesn't just heat the food faster; it also accelerates all the chemical reactions that occur in cooking. The bits of butter in a pastry crust, for example, melt faster, which means they release steam more quickly, which leads to more air between layers—in other words, a flakier crust. When roasting meats, the fat is rendered and the skin is browned more quickly, sealing in juices. The meat, because it cooks more quickly, stays moist, retaining its juicy flavor. The same is true of vegetables—the dry environment created by the fan's air circulation means the sugars caramelize more quickly, locking in moisture and providing deep, round flavor.

Although Air Fryer Toaster Oven cooking seems like new, even though professional chefs have been using it for decades due to its speed and cooking/browning features. Today these ovens are easily available to home cooks at affordable prices.

There are millions of Air Fryer Toaster Oven in private homes today, but people have had to figure out on their own how to adapt their favorite recipes, with varying°of success.

How to clean the machine

The general rule of thumb when it comes to the cleaning of the Air Fryer Toast Oven is to un-plug the fryer and allow it to cool completely.

Take out the baking pan, air fryer toast oven basket, oven rack and tray and hand wash these in warm-hot water with liquid soap. You can either use a nylon brush to clean them or a scouring pad. Do not put them in your dish washer at all. Next, clean the interior walls using a clean damp cloth or sponge with a bit of liquid soap. Do not use any abrasive materials or corrosive products as these will damage the walls. For the exterior part, use a clean damp cloth with a bit of liquid soap and it cleans up easily. Then just use a soft dry cloth to dry it completely. Avoid abrasive materials to avoid damaging the finish of the air fryer toast oven.

Every time you cook a greasy meal, clean the top interior part of the oven immediately after cooling. Doing this on a regular basis will ensure your toast oven performs very efficiently. After cleaning, use the storage cleats, located at the back of the oven to store the cord of the air fryer toast oven. Do not wrap the cord around its body as this can damage it.

For any other kind of maintenance or servicing, take your unit to authorized service personnel.

How to perfectly use an air fryer toaster oven

Before you use any function to prepare you food, note that you shouldn't use kitchen foil to cover any of the air fryer toast oven accessories as it could stop fat dripping to the pullout tray and an accumulation of fat on the kitchen foil could start a fire.

Air Fry Function

When you think air fry, think of crunchier, healthier and tastier deep frying. The Air Fry function uses cutting edge technology that involves rapid hot air circulation aided by a high-speed fan and upper heating elements to you enjoy fried food without the guilt of consuming too much oil as is the case with deep frying.

When using the Air Fryer Toast Oven, place the basket in the baking pan and place these in the lower rack position. Select Air Fry on the function dial and set the temperature according to your recipe. Turn on the ON/Oven Timer and set to the cooking time that your recipe specifies. The power light will come on and once your cooking time elapses the ringer will go off once and the oven will automatically shut itself.

Bake Function

For foods that require gentle baking such as cakes, muffins and other pastry, use the bake function. However, if you are looking for extra browning or extra crunch, use convection bake which is ideal for breads, scones, pizza, veggies and roasts.

You can make pizza on the baking pan or you can alternatively buy a pizza stone instead.

Fit your rack and baking pan into the recommended position by your recipe and select bake or convection bake. Set it to ON/ Oven Timer dial to your recipe's time. When baking pastries, you are recommended to preheat your oven for 5 minutes before the actual cook time.

The power light will come on to signify the beginning of cooking. The timer will go off once the cooking time is over and the oven will automatically turn itself off.

Toast Function

Select the toast function and place your food item at the center for even cooking.

Place your rack in the lower position and center the food items. Select toast on your function dial and select Toast/Broil to set your temperature. Turn the ON/ Toast Timer to your level of desired brownness to start toasting.

The power light will come on and once the cycle is over, the ringer will go off once before the oven automatically goes off.

Broil Function

The broil function is perfect for top browning of casseroles, gratins, pies, meats and veggies. You can use the convection broil for meats and fish as it gives a deeper browning.

Gently place the air fryer toast oven basket in the baking pan and either select Broil or Convection Broil. For the temperature, either set it to Broil/ Toast. Next, turn on the ON/ Oven Timer dial to your recipe's specification then start broiling. The power light will come on. Once the cooking is done, the timer will go off once and the oven will automatically turn off.

Note: Do not use glass dishes to broil.

Warm Function

Position the baking pan or oven rack on the lower rack position and set your temperature to warm and choose warm on your function dial. Next set your ON/Oven Timer to the desired time. The power light will come on and the ringer will go off once the time you set elapses. The oven will automatically shut itself.

Know about the Buttons and Functions

ON/ Toast Timer Dial

This allows you to select how light or dark you want your toast to be. By turning this button on, you start the toasting process for one cycle after which it will power itself off.

ON/ Oven Timer Dial

This dial sets the entire unit on apart from the toast. By turning this button on, you start the cooking cycle which when over, automatically turns itself off.

Function Dial

This is where you select your cooking method. It could either be bake, toast, broil, convection bake, convection broil or warm.

Power Light

This light comes on when the unit is in use.

Light Button

When you want to turn on the interior light, press this button with the oven on but the door closed. This automatically goes off once you open the door as it switches to power saving. The light will come back on when you close the door and food is cooking.

Oven Temperature Dial

You'll use this to set the temperature you need.

Air Fryer Toast Oven Basket

Always use the oven basket when using the air fry function for optimal results.

Pullout Tray

This is used to catch the drippings from the food you are cooking. It's removable for easier cleaning.

Cord Storage

This is located at the back of the oven and it's used for neatly tucking away the cord when the unit is off.

Oven Rack

This gives you the perfect room for baking.
Auto-shut feature the air fryer toast oven automatically turns itself off when a cooking or toasting cycle is complete.

Tips & tricks

Lightly Splash Food with Oil

You'll require your cooking splash when using your air fryer as it helps keep nourishments from adhering to the bin. Shower nourishments gently, or you could simply include a smidgen of oil.

Dry Your Food

Pat dry nourishments before cooking, particularly marinated nourishments. Doing this will forestall overabundance smoke and splattering. Nourishments that contain high-fat substances, for example, chicken bosom and wings, for the most part, store fat when cooking. Therefore, ensure you void the kept fat from the base of the air fryer on occasion.

Batch Cook

The air fryer has a little cooking limit. If you're cooking for countless individuals, you should cook in clumps.

Shake Your Container While Cooking

Open the Air Fryer at regular intervals of cooking and shake around nourishments in the bin. Chips, French fries, and other littler nourishments can pack, however, shaking around forestalls that. Pivot nourishments each 5 to 10 minutes to empower them to cook and shape well.

Distribute Evenly

Overcrowding is a no-no with the air fryer. If you need your nourishments to cook well, give it a lot of room with the goal that air can flow well. You need to appreciate the firmness of your dinners, isn't that so? Congestion keeps air from coursing over the nourishments. So, make certain to space nourishments out.

Set Fryer to Preheat Before Cooking

Preheat air fryer when it has not been used for some time. Preheat for 3-5 minutes to allow it to heat up appropriately.

Which Air Fryer toaster oven is better for me?

First of all, you read the review to know about the product. The review will give you guidelines in the case of accessories. When you are buying product, mostly brand like to offer different kinds of options for the accessories, there are some interchange the brand, and there are not.

If you buy preliminary, then you need not to buy cooker accessories. You'll get everything easier at the time of using the first time.

If you buy a any product it depends on your needs. You could get a small capacity or large capacity. It depends on your family size. In case of air fryer these depend on the amount of food made. If you buy this oven for hotel or restaurant then you purchase a large capacity. For example, you buy a 3.7L unit. It's typically a standard size and will easily make enough for 4 people.

In air fryer you give a recipe book in which all details about what you cook or fryer and what type of dish easily bake and give your idea what you can cook and get used to it at first. Air fryer provides you a safety feature. It has auto shut down and cool touch exterior. The best part of air fryer is that if you purchase Amazon, look through this entire information and read about the one with a high review and see if the advantages or disadvantages in the types of air fryer are big or small. If you want to buy air fryer for chicken or meat, then you buy a 390-400° temperature.

Chapter 2: Breakfast & brunch

Breakfast Ham Omelet

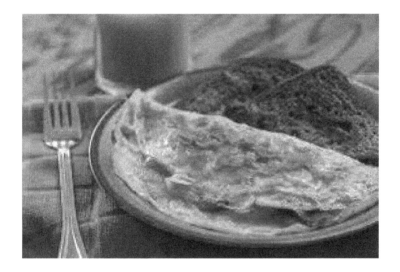

Preparation Time: 10 minutes

Cooking Time: 10 minutes

Servings: 2

Ingredients:

3 large eggs
100g ham, cut into small pieces

¼ cup milk

¾ cup mixed vegetables (white mushrooms, green onions, red pepper)

¼ cup mixed cheddar and mozzarella cheese

1 tsp. freshly chopped mixed herbs (cilantro and chives)

Salt and freshly ground pepper to taste

Directions:

Combine the eggs and milk in a medium bowl then add in the remaining ingredients apart from the cheese and mixed herbs and beat well using a fork.

Pour the egg mix into an evenly greased pan then place it in the basket of your air fryer toast oven.

Cook for roughly 10 minutes at 350°F or until done to desire. Sprinkle the cheese and mixed herbs on the omelet halfway through cook time.

Gently loosen the omelet from the sides of the pan using a spatula.

Serve hot!

Nutrition:

Calories: 411 kcal/Cal

Carbs: 14 g

Fat: 39.3 g

Protein: 28 g

Crunchy Zucchini Hash Browns

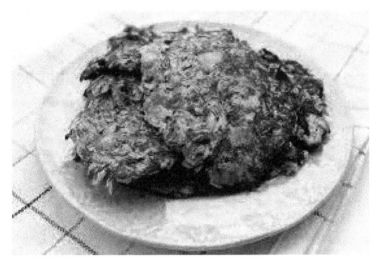

Preparation Time: 30 minutes

Cooking Time 15 minutes

Serves: 3

Ingredients:

4 medium zucchinis, peeled and grated

1 tsp. onion powder

1 tsp. garlic powder

2 tbsp. almond flour

1 ½ tsp. chili flakes

Salt and freshly ground pepper to taste

2 tsp. olive oil

Directions:

Put the grated zucchini in between layers of kitchen towel and squeeze to drain excess water. Pour 1 teaspoon of oil in a pan, preferably non-stick, over medium heat and sauté the potatoes for about 3 minutes.

Transfer the zucchini to a shallow bowl and let cool. Sprinkle it with the remaining ingredients and mix it until it forms a proper mixture.

Transfer the zucchini mix to a flat plate and pat it down to make 1 compact layer. Put in the fridge and let it sit for 20 minutes.

Set your air fryer toast oven to 360°F.

Meanwhile take out the flattened zucchini and divide into equal portions using a knife or cookie cutter.

Lightly brush your air fryer toast oven's basket with the remaining teaspoon of olive oil.

Gently place the zucchini pieces into the greased basket and fry for 12-15 minutes, flipping the hash browns halfway through.

Enjoy hot!

Nutrition

Calories: 195 kcal/Cal

Carbs: 10.4 g

Fat: 13.1 g

Protein: 9.6 g

Crunchy Hash Browns

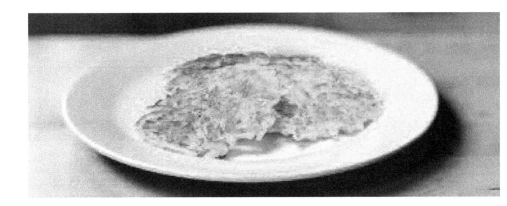

Preparation Time: 30 minutes

Cooking Time 15 minutes

Serves: 3

Ingredients:

5 medium potatoes, peeled and grated

1 tsp. onion powder

1 tsp. garlic powder

2 tbsp. corn flour

1 ½ tsp. chili flakes

Salt and freshly ground pepper to taste

2 tsp. olive oil

Directions:

Put the grated potatoes in a large bowl and cover with ice cold water and let it sit for a minute. Drain the water and repeat this step two times. (This removes the excess starch)

Pour 1 teaspoon of oil in a pan, preferably non-stick, over medium heat and sauté the potatoes for about 3 minutes. Transfer the potatoes to a shallow bowl and let cool. Sprinkle the potatoes with the remaining ingredients and mix until it combines well.

Transfer the potato mix to a flat plate and pat it down to make 1 compact layer. Put in the fridge and let it sit for 20 minutes. Set your air fryer toast oven to 360°F.

Meanwhile take out the flattened potato and divide into equal portions using a knife or cookie cutter.

Lightly brush your air fryer toast oven's basket with the remaining teaspoon of olive oil.

Gently place the potato pieces into the greased basket and fry for 12-15 minutes, flipping the hash browns halfway through. Enjoy hot!

Nutrition:

Calories: 295 kcal/Cal

Carbs: 60.9 g

Fat: 3.7 g

 Protein: 6.6 g

Meaty Breakfast Omelet

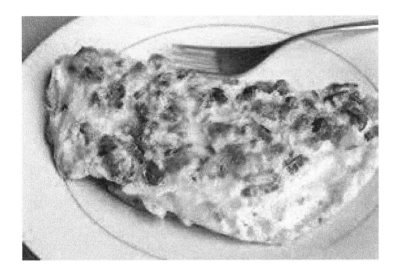

Preparation Time: 10 minutes

Cooking Time 10 minutes

Serves: 2

Ingredients:

3 large eggs

100g ham, cut into small pieces

¼ cup milk

¾ cup mixed vegetables (mushrooms, scallions, bell pepper)

¼ cup mixed cheddar and mozzarella cheese

1 tsp. mixed herbs

Salt and freshly ground pepper to taste

Directions:

Combine the eggs and milk in a medium bowl then add in the remaining ingredients apart from the cheese and mixed herbs and beat well using a fork.

Pour the egg mix into an evenly greased pan then place it in the basket of your air fryer toast oven.

Cook for roughly 10 minutes at 350°F or until done to desire. Sprinkle the cheese and mixed herbs on the omelet halfway through cook time.

Gently loosen the omelet from the sides of the pan using a spatula.

Serve hot!

Nutrition:

Calories: 278 kcal/Cal

Carbs: 1.3 g

Fat: 4.6 g

Protein: 24.1 g

Citrus Blueberry Muffins

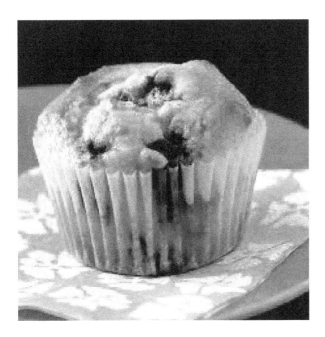

Preparation Time: 15 minutes

Cooking Time 15 minutes

Serves: 3-4

Ingredients:

2 ½ cups cake flour

½ cup sugar

¼ cup light cooking oil such as avocado oil

½ cup heavy cream

1 cup fresh blueberries

2 eggs

Zest and juice from 1 orange

1 tsp. pure vanilla extract

1 tsp. brown sugar for topping

Directions:

Start by combining the oil, heavy cream, eggs, orange juice and vanilla extract in a large bowl then set aside.

Separately combine the flour and sugar until evenly it's mixed then pour little by little into the wet ingredients.

Combine until well blended but be careful not to over-mix.

Preheat your air fryer toast oven at 320°F

Gently fold the blueberries into the batter and divide into cupcake holders, preferably, silicone cupcake holders as you won't have to grease them. Alternatively, you can use cupcake paper liners on any cupcake holders/ tray you could be having. Sprinkle the tops with the brown sugar and pop the muffins in the fryer.

Bake for about 12 minutes. Use a toothpick to check for readiness. When the muffins have evenly browned and an inserted toothpick comes out clean, they are ready.

Take out the muffins and let cool.

Enjoy!

Nutrition:

Calories: 289 kcal/Cal,

Carbs: 12.8 g

Fat: 32 g

Protein: 21.1 g

PB &J Donuts

Preparation Time: 15 minutes

Cooking Time 12 minutes

Serves: 4

Ingredients:

For the Donuts:

1 ¼ cups all-purpose flour

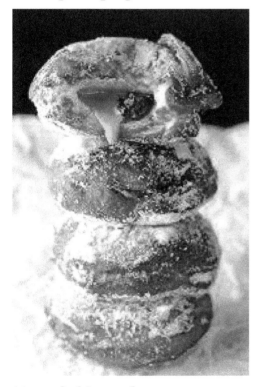

½ tsp. baking soda

½ tsp. baking powder

1/3 cup sugar

½ cup buttermilk

1 large egg

1 tsp. pure vanilla extract

3 tbsp. unsalted, melted and divided into 2+1

¾ tsp. salt

For the Glaze:

2 tbsp. milk

½ cup powdered sugar

2 tbsp. smooth peanut butter

Sea salt to taste

For the Filling:

½ cup strawberry or blueberry jelly

Directions:

Whisk together all the dry ingredients for the donut in a large bowl.

Separately combine the egg, buttermilk, melted butter and vanilla extract.

Create a small well at the center of the dry ingredients and pour in the egg mixture. Use a fork to combine the ingredients then finish off with a spatula.

Place the dough on a floured surface and knead the dough. It will start out sticky but as you knead, it's going to come together.

Roll out the dough to make a ¾ inch thick circle. Use a cookie cutter, or the top part of a cup to cut the dough into rounds.

Place the donuts on a parchment paper and then into your air fryer toast oven. You may have to cook in batches depending on the size of your unit.

Cook for 12 minutes at 350°F.

Use a pastry bag or squeeze bottle to fill the donuts with jelly.

Combine the glaze ingredients and drizzle on top of the donuts.

Enjoy!

Nutrition:

Calories: 430 kcal/Cal

Carbs: 66.8 g

Fat: 14.6 g

Protein: 9.1 g

Breakfast Baked Apple

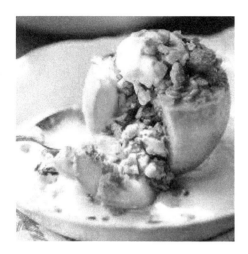

Preparation Time: 10 minutes

Cooking Time 20 minutes

Serves: 2

Ingredients:

1 apple

2 tbsp. raisins

2 tbsp. walnuts, chopped

¼ tsp. nutmeg

¼ tsp. ground cinnamon

1 ½ tsp. margarine

¼ cup water

Directions:

Start by setting your air fryer toast oven to 350°F.

Cut the apple in half and gently spoon out some of the flesh.

Place the apple halves on your air fryer toast ovens frying pan.

Mix the raisins, walnuts, nutmeg, cinnamon and margarine in a bowl and divide equally between the apple halves.

Pour the water into the pan and cook for 20 minutes.

Enjoy!

Nutrition:

Calories: 161 kcal/Cal

Carbs: 23.7 g

Fat: 7.8 g

Protein: 2.5g

Sunny Side up Egg Tarts

Preparation Time: 15 minutes

Cooking Time 20 minutes

Serves: 2

Ingredients:

4 eggs

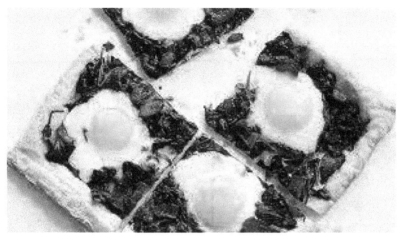

¾ cup shredded Gruyere cheese (or preferred cheese)

1 sheet of puff pastry

Minced chives for topping

Directions:

Start by flouring a clean surface then gently roll out your sheet of puff pastry and divide it into four equal squares.

If you have a small air fryer toast oven, start with two squares but if it's big enough, go ahead and place the squares on the basket and cook for about 8-10 minutes or until they turn golden brown.

Whilst still in the basket, gently make an indentation at the center of each square and sprinkle 2-4 tablespoons of shredded cheese in the well then crack an egg on top.

Cook for 5-10 minutes or to desired doneness.

Remove from air fryer toast oven, sprinkle with chives and you are ready to eat!

Nutrition:

Calories: 403 kcal/Cal

Carbs: 10.8 g

Fat: 29.4 g

Protein: 24.6 g

Healthy Spinach Scramble

Preparation Time: 8 minutes

Cooking Time 30 minutes

Serves: 1

Ingredients:

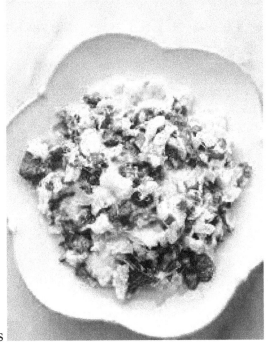

3 egg whites

1 cup (packed) spinach

1 onion, chopped

2 tbsp. extra virgin olive oil

½ tsp. onion powder

½ tsp. garlic powder

1 tsp. turmeric powder

Ground pepper to taste

Directions:

Preheat your air fryer toast oven to 350°F.

Beat the egg whites and oil in a large bowl. Add in the fresh ingredients and mix until well combined then set the bowl aside.

Lightly grease your air fryer toast oven's frying pan and transfer the egg mixture into the pan.

Cook in the fryer for about 10 minutes or until done to desire. Serve hot.

Nutrition:

 Calories: 285 kcal/Cal

Carbs: 12.3 g

Fat: 21.6 g

Protein: 13 g

Healthy Vegan Scramble

Preparation Time: 8 minutes

Cooking Time 30 minutes

Serves: 3

Ingredients:

2 large potatoes, cut into cubes

1 tofu block, cut into cubes

1 broccoli, divided into florets

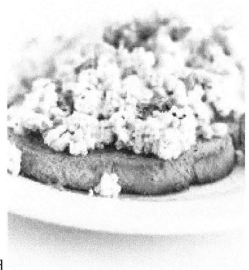

1 large onion, chopped

2 tbsp. dark soy sauce

2 tbsp. extra virgin olive oil, divided into 1+1

½ tsp. onion powder

½ tsp. garlic powder

1 tsp. turmeric powder

Ground pepper to taste

Directions:

Start by marinating the tofu in 1 tablespoon of olive oil onion, garlic, turmeric and onion powders then set aside.

Drizzle the potatoes with the remaining tablespoon of olive oil and toss with pepper and cook in the air fryer toast oven for 15 minutes at 400°F. Halfway through cook time, toss the potatoes to allow even cooking.

Toss the potatoes once more then mix in the marinated tofu, reserving the leftover liquid and cook for another 15 minutes at 370°F.

Toss the broccoli florets in the leftover marinade. If it's too little, drizzle with some soy sauce and toss to ensure all the florets are evenly covered.

When the potato-tofu mixture has 5 minutes of cooking time left, add in the broccoli.

Serve hot.

Nutrition:

Calories: 319 kcal/Cal

Carbs: 50.4 g

Fat: 10.9 g,

Protein: 8 g

Ham and Cheese sandwich

Preparation Time: 15 minutes

Cooking Time 20 minutes

Serves: 2

Ingredients:

2 eggs

4 slices of bread of choice

4 slices turkey

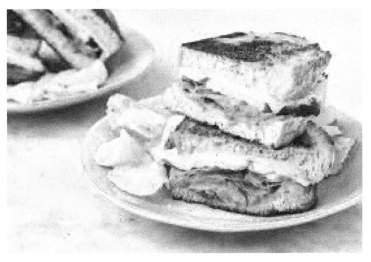

4 slices ham

6 tbsp. half and half cream

2 tsp. melted butter

4 slices Swiss cheese

¼ tsp. pure vanilla extract

Powdered sugar and raspberry jam for serving

Directions:

Mix the eggs, vanilla and cream in a bowl and set aside.

Make a sandwich with the bread layered with cheese slice, turkey, ham, cheese slice and the top slice of bread to make two sandwiches. Gently press on the sandwiches to somewhat flatten them.

Set your air fryer toast oven to 350°F.

Spread out kitchen aluminum foil and cut it about the same size as the sandwich and spread the melted butter on the surface of the foil.

Dip the sandwich in the egg mixture and let it soak for about 20 seconds on each side. Repeat this for the other sandwich.

Place the soaked sandwiches on the prepared foil sheets then place on the basket in your fryer.

Cook for 12 minutes then flip the sandwiches and brush with the remaining butter and cook for another 5 minutes or until well browned.

Place the cooked sandwiched on a plate and top with the powdered sugar and serve with a small bowl of raspberry jam. Enjoy!

Nutrition:

Calories: 735 kcal/Cal

Carbs: 13.4 g

Fat: 47.9 g

Protein: 40.8 g

Healthy Squash

Preparation Time: 10 minutes

Cooking Time: 25 minutes

Servings: 4

Ingredients:

2 lbs. yellow squash, cut into half-moons

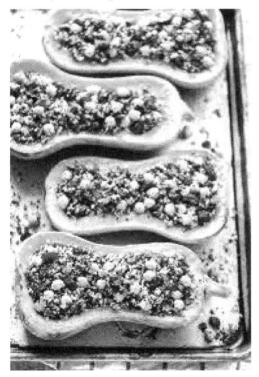

1 tsp. Italian seasoning

¼ tsp. pepper

1 tbsp. olive oil

¼ tsp. salt

Directions:

Add all ingredients into the large bowl and toss well.

Preheat the air fryer to 400°F.

Add squash mixture into the air fryer basket and cook for 10 minutes.

Shake basket and cook for another 10 minutes.

Shake once again and cook for 5 minutes more.

Nutrition:

Calories: 70 kcal/Cal

Fat: 4 g

Carbohydrates: 7 g

Sugar: 4 g

Protein: 2 g

Cholesterol: 1 mg

Spinach Frittata

Preparation Time: 10 minutes

Cooking Time: 8 minutes

Servings: 6

Ingredients:

8 eggs

1/4 cup mushrooms, sliced 1 tbsp. olive oil

1 cups spinach

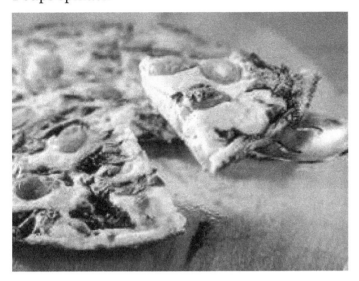

1 tbsp. curry powder 1/4 cup onion, diced Pepper

Salt

Directions:

Preheat the air fryer to 325°F.

Heat the oil in a pan over medium-high heat.

Add onion and mushrooms to the pan and sauté for 5-8 minutes.

Add spinach and cook for 2 minutes.

In a large bowl, whisk eggs, curry powder, pepper, and salt.

Transfer pan mixture into the air fryer baking dish. Pour egg mixture over vegetables and stir well.

Place dish in the air fryer and cook for 8 minutes or until eggs are set

Serve and enjoy.

Nutrition:

Calories: 116 kcal/Cal

Fat: 8 g

Carbohydrates: 2 g

Sugar: 1 g

Protein: 8 g

Cholesterol: 218 mg

Lemon Dill Scallops

Preparation Time: 10 minutes

Cooking Time: 5 minutes

Servings: 4

Ingredients:

1 lb. scallops

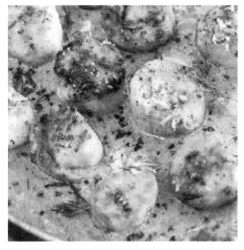

2 tsp. olive oil

1 tsp. dill, chopped

1 tbsp. fresh lemon juice Pepper

Salt

Directions:

Add scallops into the bowl and toss with oil, dill, lemon juice, pepper, and salt.

Add scallops into the air fryer basket and cook at 360°F for 5 minutes.

Serve and enjoy.

Nutrition:

Calories: 121 kcal/Cal

Fat: 3.2 g

Carbohydrates: 2.9 g

Sugar: 0.1 g

Protein: 19 g

Cholesterol: 37 mg

Herb Mushrooms

Preparation Time: 10 minutes

Cooking Time: 12 minutes

Servings: 2

Ingredients:

10 mushrooms, stems remove
1 tbsp. dill, chopped

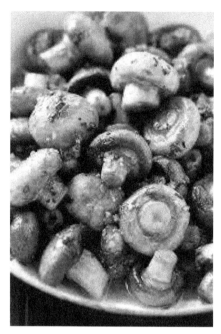

1 tbsp. olive oil 1 tbsp. parmesan cheese, grated

½ tbsp. oregano

½ tsp. dried basil

Pepper and salt

Directions:

Add mushrooms into the bowl and toss with oil, oregano, basil, pepper, and salt.

Add mushrooms into the air fryer basket and cook at 360 F for 6 minutes.

Add dill and cheese and toss well and cook for 6 minutes more.

Serve and enjoy.

Nutrition:

Calories: 87 kcal/Cal

Fat: 7 g

Carbohydrates: 4 g

Sugar: 1 g

Protein: 3 g

Cholesterol: 0 mg

Easy & Tasty Salsa Chicken

Preparation Time: 10 minutes

Cooking Time: 30 minutes

Servings: 4

Ingredients:

1 lb. chicken thighs, boneless and skinless

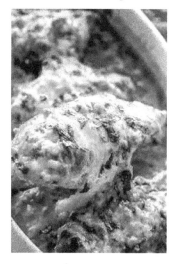

1 cup salsa

Pepper Salt

Directions:

Preheat the air fryer to 350°F.

Place chicken thighs into the air fryer baking dish and season with pepper and salt. Top with salsa.

Place in the air fryer and cook for 30 minutes.

Serve and enjoy.

Nutrition:

Calories: 233 kcal/Cal

Fat: 8 g

Carbohydrates: 4 g

Sugar: 2 g

Protein: 33 g

Cholesterol: 101 mg

Fish and Chips

Preparation Time: 10 minutes

Cooking Time: 12 minutes

Servings: 2

Ingredients:

2 medium cod fillets, skinless and boneless

Salt and black pepper to the taste

¼ cup margarine milk

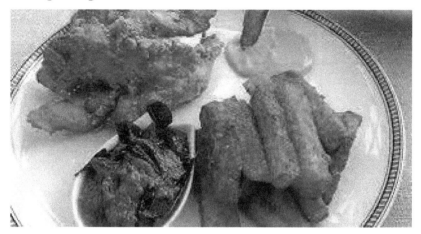

3 cups kettle chips, cooked

Directions:

In a bowl, mix fish with salt, pepper and margarine milk, toss and leave aside for 5 minutes.

Put chips in your food processor, crush them and spread them on a plate.

Add fish and press well on all sides.

Transfer fish to your air fryer's basket and cook at 400 °F for 12 minutes.

Serve hot for lunch.

Nutrition:

Calories: 113 kcal/Cal

 Fat: 8.2 g

Carbohydrates: 0.3 g

Sugar: 0.2 g

Protein: 5.4 g

Cholesterol: 18 mg

Delicious Beef Cubes

Preparation Time: 10 minutes

Cooking Time: 12 minutes

Servings: 4

Ingredients:

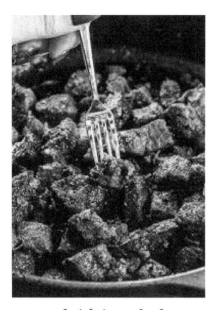

1-pound sirloin, cubed

16 ounces jarred pasta sauce

1 and ½ cups breadcrumbs

2 tbsp. olive oil

½ tsp. marjoram, dried

White rice, already cooked for serving

Directions:

In a bowl, mix beef cubes with pasta sauce and toss well.

In another bowl, mix breadcrumbs with marjoram and oil and stir well.

Dip beef cubes in this mix, place them in your air fryer and cook at 360 °F for 12 minutes.

Divide among plates and serve with white rice on the side.

Nutrition:

Calories: 113 kcal/Cal

Fat: 8.2 g

Carbohydrates: 0.3 g

Sugar: 0.2 g

Protein: 5.4 g

Cholesterol: 18 mg

Pasta Salad

Preparation Time: 10 minutes

Cooking Time: 12 minutes

Servings: 6

Ingredients:

1 zucchini, sliced in half and roughly chopped

1 orange bell pepper, roughly chopped

1 green bell pepper, roughly chopped

1 red onion, roughly chopped

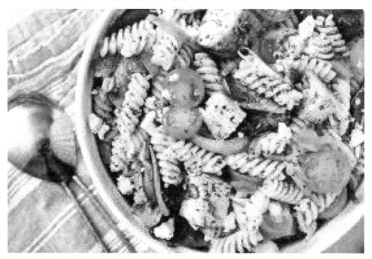

4 ounces' brown mushrooms, halved

Salt and black pepper to the taste

1 tsp. Italian seasoning

1-pound penne rig ate, already cooked

1 cup cherry tomatoes, halved

½ cup Kalamata olive, pitted and halved

¼ cup olive oil

3 tbsp. balsamic vinegar

2 tbsp. basil, chopped

Directions:

In a bowl, mix zucchini with mushrooms, orange bell pepper, green bell pepper, red onion, salt, pepper, Italian seasoning and oil, toss well, transfer to preheated air fryer at 380°F and cook them for 12 minutes.

In a large salad bowl, mix pasta with cooked veggies, cherry tomatoes, olives, vinegar and basil, toss and serve for lunch.

Nutrition:

Calories: 113 kcal/Cal

Fat: 8.2 g

Carbohydrates: 0.3 g

Sugar: 0.2 g

Protein: 5.4 g

Cholesterol: 18 mg

Chapter 3: Lunch Recipes

Garlicky Fish Fingers

Preparation Time: 10 minutes

Cooking Time: 10 minutes

Servings: 4

Ingredients:

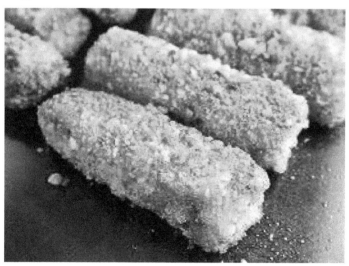

2/3 lb. white fish, boneless, cut into fingers

½ tsp. salt

2 tbsp. lemon juice

½ tsp. turmeric powder

½ tsp. red chili flakes

2 tsp. mixed dried herbs, divided

2 tsp. garlic powder, divided

½ tsp. crushed black pepper

1 tsp. ginger garlic paste

2 tbsp. flour

1 tsp. rice flour

2 tsp. corn flour

2 egg

¼ tsp. baking soda

1 cup breadcrumbs

Oil for brushing

Directions:

Beat eggs with lemon juice and garlic paste in a shallow bowl, mix corn flour with rice flour, black pepper, garlic powder, herbs, chili flakes, turmeric powder, salt, and baking soda in another tray. Coat the fish fingers with flour mixture, then dip in the egg and coat with the breadcrumbs. Place the fish fingers in the Air Fryer basket. Spray the fingers with cooking oil. Set the basket inside the Air Fryer toaster oven and close the lid. Select the Air Fry mode at 356°F temperature for 10 minutes. Serve warm.

Nutrition

Calories: 279 kcal/Cal

Protein: 32.9g

Carbs: 28.1g

Fat: 15.7g

Korean Barbeque Beef

Preparation Time: 15 minutes

Cooking Time: 30 minutes

Servings: 4

Ingredients:

1 Lb. flank steak

1/4 Cup corn starch

1 Tablespoon Pompeian oil

1/2 Cup soy sauce

1/2 Cup brown sugar

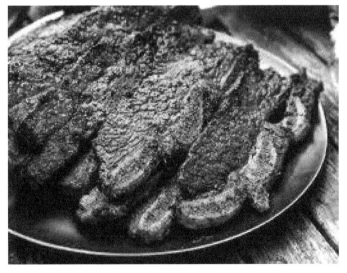

2 Tablespoons Pompeian while vinegar

1 Tablespoon garlic (crushed)

½ Tablespoon sesame seeds

1 Tablespoon corn starch

1 Tablespoon water

Direction

The steak should be sliced into thin pieces and rubbed with corn starch and oil. The air fryer toaster oven should be preheated at 390°F for 5 min. The basket should be covered by aluminum foil. The steaks are placed in the basket and heated for 20 min with intermittent flipping. In the meantime, all other ingredients are heated in a pan except water and cornstarch in medium heat to form the sauce. The sauce should be heated until reduced to half. The sauce should be poured over the steak and served with green beans and cooked rice.

Nutrition

Calories: 487 kcal/Cal

Fat: 10 g

Carbs: 32 g

Protein: 39g

Beef Burgers

Preparation Time: 5 minutes

Cooking Time: 15 minutes

Servings: 4

Ingredients

4 Ground beef patties

¼ Tablespoon black pepper

4 Slices sharp cheddar cheese

1/2 Cup onion (sliced)

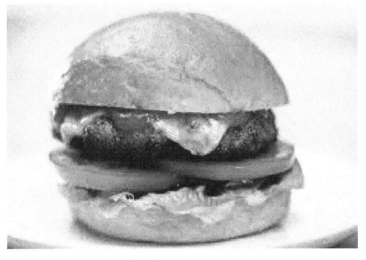

1/2 Cup tomato (sliced)

1 Tablespoon pickles

4 Leaves lettuce

½ Tablespoon mustard

4 hamburger Buns

Directions

The beef patties are rubbed with black pepper. The air fryer toaster oven should be preheated at 375F for 5 min. The basket should be covered by aluminum foil. The patties are placed in the basket and heated for 10 min with intermittent flipping. One slice of cheese is placed on each patty and heated for another 2 min. One cooked patty is placed on one bun to which are added lettuce leaves, pickles, onion and mustard and covered by another bun. Thus, the burger gets ready to be served.

Nutrition

Calories: 240 kcal/Cal

Fat: 6g

Carbs: 11 g

Protein: 16g

Chicken Pot Pie

Preparation Time: 10 minutes

Cooking Time: 17 minutes

Servings: 6

Ingredients

2 tbsp. olive oil

1-pound chicken breast cubed
1 tbsp. garlic powder

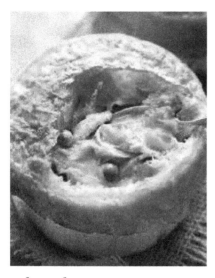

1 tbsp. thyme

1 tbsp. pepper

1 cup chicken broth

12 oz. bag frozen mixed vegetables

4 large potatoes cubed

10 oz. Can cream of chicken soup

1 cup heavy cream

1 pie crust

1 egg 1 tbsp. water

Directions

Hit Sauté on the Instant Pot Duo Crispy and add chicken and olive oil.

Sauté chicken for 5 minutes then stir in spices.

Pour in the broth along with vegetables and cream of chicken soup

Put on the pressure-cooking lid and seal it.

Hit the "Pressure Button" and select 10 minutes of cooking time, then press "Start."

Once the Instant Pot Duo beeps, do a quick release and remove its lid.

Remove the lid and stir in cream.

Hit sauté and cook for 2 minutes.

Enjoy!

Nutrition

Calories: 568 kcal/Cal

Fat: 31.1g

Carbohydrates: 50.8g

Fiber: 3.9g

Protein: 23.4g

Chicken Casserole

Preparation Time: 10 Minutes

Cooking Time: 9 minutes

Servings: 6

Ingredients

3 cup chicken, shredded

12 oz. bag egg noodles

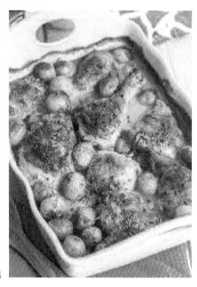

1/2 large onion

1/2 cup chopped carrots

1/4 cup frozen peas

1/4 cup frozen broccoli pieces

2 stalks celery chopped

5 cup chicken broth

1 teaspoon garlic powder

Salt and pepper to taste

1 cup cheddar cheese, shredded

1 package French's onions

1/4 c sour cream

1 can cream of chicken and mushroom soup

Directions

Add chicken, broth, black pepper, salt, garlic powder, vegetables, and egg noodles to the Instant Pot Duo.

Put on the pressure-cooking lid and seal it.

Hit the "Pressure Button" and select 4 minutes of cooking time, then press "Start."

Once the Instant Pot Duo beeps, do a quick release and remove its lid.

Stir in cheese, 1/3 of French's onions, can of soup and sour cream.

Mix well and spread the remaining onion top.

Put on the Air Fryer lid and seal it.

Hit the "Air fryer Button" and select 5 minutes of cooking time, then press "Start."

Once the Instant Pot Duo beeps, remove its lid.

Serve.

Nutrition

Calories: 494 kcal/Cal

Fat: 19.1g

Carbohydrates: 29g

Fiber: 2.6g

Protein: 48.9g

Ranch Chicken Wings

Preparation Time: 10 minutes

Cooking Time: 35 minutes

Servings: 6

Ingredients

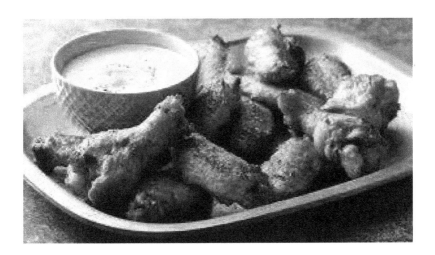

12 chicken wings

1 tablespoon olive oil

1 cup chicken broth

1/4 cup butter

1/2 cup Red Hot Sauce

1/4 teaspoon Worcestershire sauce

1 tablespoon white vinegar

1/4 teaspoon cayenne pepper

1/8 teaspoon garlic powder

Seasoned salt to taste

Ranch dressing for dipping Celery for garnish

Directions

Set the Air Fryer Basket in the Instant Pot Duo and pour the broth in it.

Spread the chicken wings in the basket and put on the pressure-cooking lid.

Hit the "Pressure Button" and select 10 minutes of cooking time, then press "Start."

Meanwhile, prepare the sauce and add butter, vinegar, cayenne pepper, garlic powder, Worcestershire sauce, and hot sauce in a small saucepan.

Stir cook this sauce for 5 minutes on medium heat until it thickens.

Once the Instant Pot Duo beeps, do a quick release and remove its lid.

Remove the wings and empty the Instant Pot Duo.

Toss the wings with oil, salt, and black pepper.

Set the Air Fryer Basket in the Instant Pot Duo and arrange the wings in it.

Put on the Air Fryer lid and seal it.

Hit the "Air Fryer Button" and select 20 minutes of cooking time, then press "Start."

Once the Instant Pot beeps, remove its lid.

Transfer the wings to the sauce and mix well.

Serve.

Nutrition

Calories: 414

Fat: 31.6g

Carbohydrates 11.2g

Fiber: 0.3g

Protein: 20.4g

Tofu Sushi Burrito

Preparation Time: 5 minutes
Cooking Time: 15 minutes
Servings: 2

Ingredients

¼ block extra firm tofu, pressed and sliced

1 tbsp. low-sodium soy sauce

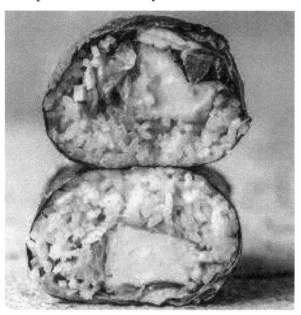

¼ tsp. ground ginger

¼ tsp. garlic powder

Sriracha sauce, to taste

2 cups cooked sushi rice

2 sheets nori

Filling:

¼ avocado, sliced

3 tbsp mango, sliced

1 green onion, finely chopped

2 tbsp. pickled ginger

2 tbsp. panko breadcrumbs

Directions

Whisk ginger, garlic, soy sauce, sriracha sauce, and tofu in a large bowl.

Let them marinate for 10 minutes then transfer them to the air fryer basket.

Return the fryer basket to the air fryer and cook on air fry mode for 15 minutes at 370°F.

Toss the tofu cubes after 8 minutes then resume cooking.

Spread a nori sheet on a work surface and top it with a layer of sushi rice.

Place tofu and half of the other filling ingredients over the rice.

Roll the sheet tightly to secure the filling inside.

Repeat the same steps to make another sushi roll.

Enjoy!

Nutrition

Calories: 372 kcal/Cal

Fat: 11.8 g

Carbohydrates: 45.8 g

Fiber: 0.6 g

Protein: 34 g

Rosemary Brussels Sprouts

Preparation Time: 5 minutes

Cooking Time: 13 minutes

Servings: 2

Ingredients

3 tbsp. olive oil

2 garlic cloves, minced

½ tsp. salt

¼ tsp. pepper

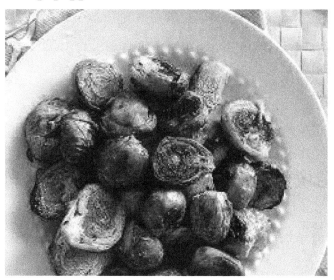

1 lb. Brussels sprouts, trimmed and halved

½ cup panko breadcrumbs

1 ½ tsp. fresh rosemary, minced

Directions

Let your air fryer preheat at 350°F.

Mix oil, garlic, salt, and pepper in a bowl and heat for 30 seconds in the microwave.

Add 2 tablespoons of this mixture to the Brussels sprouts in a bowl and mix well to coat.

Spread the sprouts in the air fryer basket.

Return the fryer basket to the air fryer and cook on air fry mode for 5 minutes at 220°F.

Toss the sprouts well and continue air frying for 8 minutes more.

Mix the remaining oil mixture with rosemary and breadcrumbs in a bowl.

Spread this mixture over the Brussels sprouts and return the basket to the fryer.

Air fry them for 5 minutes.

Enjoy.

Nutrition

Calories: 246 kcal/Cal

Fat: 7.4 g

Carbohydrates: 9.4 g

Fiber: 2.7 g

Protein: 37.2 g

Peach-Bourbon Wings

Preparation Time: 5 minutes

Cooking Time: 14 minutes

Servings: 8

Ingredients

½ cup peach preserves

1 tbsp. brown sugar

1 garlic clove, minced

¼ tsp. salt

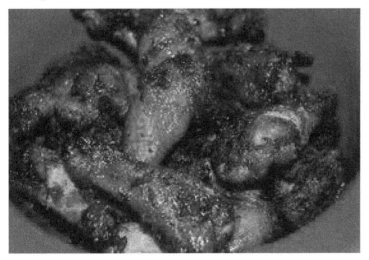

2 tbsp. white vinegar

2 tbsp. bourbon

1 tsp. cornstarch

1½ tsp. water

2 lbs. chicken wings

Directions

Let your air fryer preheat at 400°F.

Add salt, garlic, and brown sugar to a food processor and blend well until smooth.

Transfer this mixture to a saucepan and add bourbon, peach preserves, and vinegar.

Stir cook this mixture to a boil then reduce heat to a simmer. Cook for 6 minutes until the mixture thickens.

Mix cornstarch with water and pour this mixture in the saucepan.

Stir cook for 2 minutes until it thickens. Keep ¼ cup of this sauce aside.

Place the wings in the air fryer basket and brush them with prepared sauce.

Return the fryer basket to the air fryer and cook on air fry mode for 6 minutes at 350°F.

Flip the wings and brush them again with the sauce.

Air fry the wings for another 8 minutes.

Serve with reserved sauce.

Nutrition

Calories: 293 kcal/Cal

Fat: 16 g

Carbohydrates: 5.2 g

Fiber: 1.9 g

Protein: 34.2 g

Reuben Calzones

Preparation Time: 5 minutes

Cooking Time: 12 minutes

Servings: 4

Ingredients

1 tube (13.8 ounces) refrigerated pizza crust

4 slices Swiss cheese

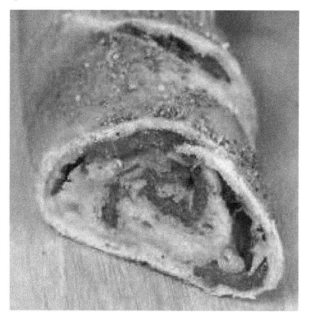

1 cup sauerkraut, rinsed and well drained

½ lb. corned beef, sliced & cooked

Directions

Let your air fryer preheat at 400°F. Grease the air fryer basket with cooking oil.

Spread the pizza crust on a lightly floured surface into a 12-inch square.

Slice the crust into four smaller squares.

Place one slice of cheese, ¼ of the sauerkraut, and 1 slice corned beef over each square diagonally.

Fold the squares in half diagonally to form a triangle and pinch the edges together.

Place 2 triangles in the air fryer basket at a time and spray them with cooking oil.

Return the fryer basket to the air fryer and cook on air fry mode for 12 minutes at 350°F.

Air fry the remaining calzone triangles.

Enjoy with fresh salad.

Nutrition

Calories: 604 kcal/Cal

Fat: 30.6 g

Carbohydrates: 31.4 g

 Fiber: 0.2 g

Protein: 54.6 g

Braised Pork

Preparation Time: 40 minutes

Cooking Time: 40 minutes

Servings: 2

Ingredients

1-pound pork loin roast, boneless and cubed

2 tablespoons butter, melted and divided

Salt and black pepper, to taste

1 cup chicken stock

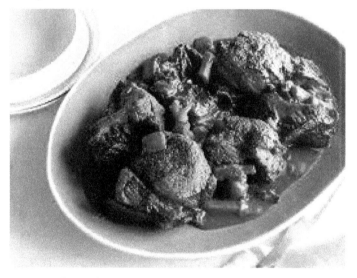

¼ cup dry white wine

1 clove garlic, minced

½ teaspoon thyme, chopped

½ thyme sprig

1 bay leaf

¼ yellow onion, chopped

1 tablespoon white flour

¼ pound red grapes

Directions

Season pork cubes with salt and pepper. Rub with half the melted butter and put in the air fryer. Cook at 370F for 8 minutes.

Meanwhile, heat a pan on the stove with 2 tablespoons of butter over medium heat. Add onion and garlic, and stir-fry for 2 minutes.

Add bay leaf, flour, thyme, salt, pepper, stock, and wine. Mix well. Bring to a simmer and take off the heat.

Add grapes and pork cubes. Cook in the air fryer at 360°F for 30 minutes.

Serve.

Nutrition

Calories: 320 kcal/Cal

Fat: 4 g

Carbohydrates: 29 g

Protein: 38 g

Lean Beef with Green Onions

Preparation Time: 10 minutes

Cooking Time: 20 minutes

Servings: 2

Ingredients

½ cup green onion, chopped

½ cup soy sauce

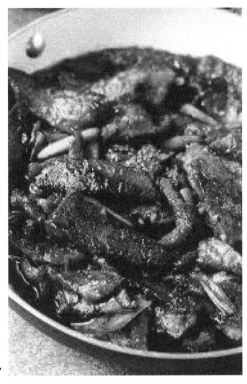

¼ cup water

2 tablespoons brown sugar

2 tablespoons sesame seeds

2 cloves garlic, minced

½ teaspoon black pepper

½ pound lean beef

Directions

In a bowl, mix the onion with water, soy sauce, garlic, sugar, sesame seeds, and pepper. Whisk and add meat. Marinate for 10 minutes.

Drain beef. Preheat the air fryer to 390F, then cook beef for 20 minutes.

Serve.

Nutrition

Calories: 329 kcal/Cal

Fat: 8 g

Carbohydrates: 26 g

Protein: 22 g

Lamb Shanks

Preparation Time: 10 minutes

Cooking Time: 45 minutes

Servings: 2

Ingredients

2 lamb shanks

½ yellow onion, chopped

½ tablespoon olive oil

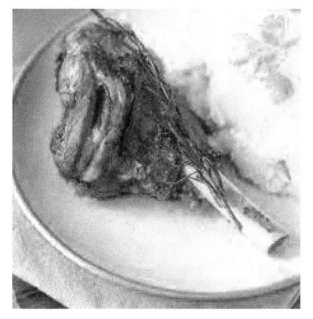

2 teaspoons crushed coriander seeds

1 tablespoon white flour

2 bay leaves

1 teaspoon honey

2 ½ ounces dry sherry

1 ¼ cups chicken stock

Salt and pepper, to taste

Directions

Season the lamb shanks with salt and pepper. Rub with half of the oil and cook in the air fryer at 360F for 10 minutes.

Heat up a pan with the rest of the oil over medium-high heat. Add onion and coriander. Stir and cook for 5 minutes.

Add salt, pepper, bay leaves, honey, stock, sherry, and flour. Bring to a simmer while stirring, then add the lamb. Mix well. Cook in the air fryer at 360°F for 30 minutes.

Serve.

Nutrition

Calories: 283 kcal/Cal

Fat: 4 g

Carbohydrates: 17 g

Protein: 26 g

Beef and Cheese Enchiladas

Preparation Time: 10 minutes

Cooking Time: 20 minutes

Servings: 4

Ingredients:

1 Lb. ground beef

1 Tablespoon taco seasoning

8 Gluten free tortillas

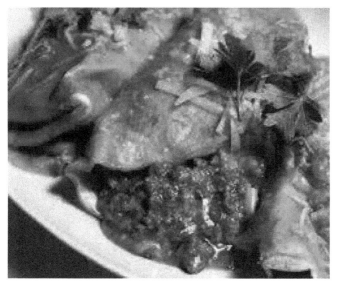

1 Can black beans (rinsed)

1 Can diced tomatoes

1 Can chopped green chilies

1 Cup Mexican cheese (shredded)

1 Can red Enchilada sauce

1 Cup fresh cilantro (chopped)

½ Cup sour Cream

Directions

The ground beef should be cooked in a frying pan till brown. The cooked beef should be covered by taco seasonings. The tomatoes, beans, chilies should be added to the beef and mixed thoroughly. The mixture is used to cover the tortillas followed by enchiladas sauce. The air fryer should be preheated at 355°F for 5 min. The tortillas are placed in the basket and topping is done by cheese. They are heated for 6 min with intermittent flipping. The cooked tortillas are removed from the basket, topped with cilantro and cream and served hot.

Nutrition

Calories: 454 kcal/Cal

Fat: 8 g

Carbs: 40 g

Protein: 26 g

Asian Style Vegetable with Beef

Preparation Time: 10 minutes

Cooking Time: 10 minutes

Servings: 4

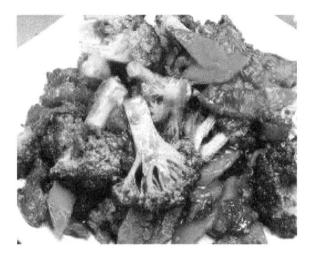

Ingredients:

1 lb. sirloin steak

2 Tablespoons corn starch

1 Red pepper (sliced)

½ Yellow onion (sliced)

1 Tablespoon garlic (minced)

2 Tablespoons ginger (grated)

1/2 Cup soy sauce

1 Tablespoon sesame oil

1/4 Cup rice vinegar

1/3 Cup brown sugar

1/4 Cup water

Directions

The steak should be cut into strips. All the ingredients are mixed thoroughly to form a mixture to marinade. The steak strips are placed inside a zip bag to which is added the mixture is added and kept in the refrigerator overnight to marinade. The steak pieces are removed from the bag by tongs and placed in the cutting board for 5 min. The air fryer toaster oven should be preheated at 390 F for 5 min. The basket should be covered by aluminum foil. The steaks are placed in the basket and heated for 6 min with intermittent flipping. The cooked steaks are removed from the basket, garnished with scallions and sesame seeds and served hot.

Nutrition

Calories: 289 kcal/Cal

Fat: 7 g

Carbs: 27 g

Protein: 31 g

Preparation Time: 10 minutes

Cooking Time: 10 minutes

Servings: 4

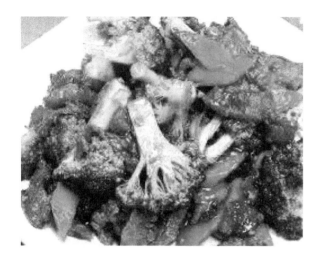

Ingredients:

1 lb. sirloin steak

2 Tablespoons corn starch

1 Red pepper (sliced)

½ Yellow onion (sliced)

1 Tablespoon garlic (minced)

2 Tablespoons ginger (grated)

1/2 Cup soy sauce

1 Tablespoon sesame oil

1/4 Cup rice vinegar

1/3 Cup brown sugar

1/4 Cup water

Directions

The steak should be cut into strips. All the ingredients are mixed thoroughly to form a mixture to marinade. The steak strips are placed inside a zip bag to which is added the mixture is added and kept in the refrigerator overnight to marinade. The steak pieces are removed from the bag by tongs and placed in the cutting board for 5 min. The air fryer toaster oven should be preheated at 390 F for 5 min. The basket should be covered by aluminum foil. The steaks are placed in the basket and heated for 6 min with intermittent flipping. The cooked steaks are removed from the basket, garnished with scallions and sesame seeds and served hot.

Nutrition

Calories: 289 kcal/Cal

Fat: 7 g

Carbs: 27 g

Protein: 31 g

Beef Meatballs

Preparation Time: 10 minutes

Cooking Time: 15 minutes

Servings: 4

Ingredients:

1 Lb. lean ground beef

1 Tablespoon pizza seasoning

1 Tablespoon minced garlic

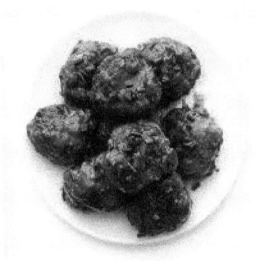

1 Tablespoon dried onion (minced)

1 Egg

¼ Tablespoon salt

1 Cup marinara sauce

1/3 Cup parmesan (shredded)

¼ Cup Mozzarella cheese

Directions

All the listed ingredients should be mixed except the marinara sauce and mozzarella cheese. The mixture should be made into 12 meatballs. The air fryer should be preheated at 350°F for 5 min. The steak strips are placed inside a zip bag to which is added the mixture is added and kept in the refrigerator overnight to marinade. The steak pieces are removed from the bag by tongs and placed in the cutting board for 5 min. The basket should be covered by aluminum foil. The steaks are placed in the basket and 6 min with intermittent flipping. The cooked steaks are removed from the basket, garnished with scallions and sesame seeds and served hot.

Nutrition

Calories: 289 kcal/Cal

Fat: 7 g

Carbs: 27 g

Protein: 31 g

Guacamole

Preparation Time: 10 minutes

Cooking Time: 20 minutes

Servings: 4

Ingredients:

1 Egg

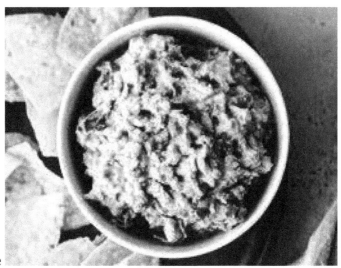

1 Egg white

1/3 Cup almond flour

2 Cup panko

1 Tablespoon olive oil

Guacamole

3 Avocado (ripe)

1/3 Cup onion (chopped)

1/3 Cup cilantro (chopped)

1 Lemon juice

¼ Tablespoon salt

¼ Tablespoon pepper

1 Tablespoon cumin

8 Table spoon almond flour

Directions

The whole ingredients for guacamole should be mixed in a bowl and the mixture should be placed in the refrigerator for thickening for 2 hours. The guacamole is taken out from the refrigerator and made into balls and placed on a baking tray. The balls are again put in the refrigerator for 6 hours or overnight. Three bowls are taken and one of which contains a beaten egg, flour in the second and panko crumbs in the third. The guacamole balls are rubbed with oil and coated with flour, egg and finally panko. The air fryer toaster oven should be preheated at 390°F for 5 min. The balls are placed in the basket and heated for 8 min with intermittent flipping. The balls are removed from the basket when they become brown. The potatoes are placed in a bowl and served with sauce.

Nutrition

Calories: 179 kcal/Cal

Fat: 13 g

Carbs: 17 g

Protein: 6 g

Lamb Chops and Horseradish Sauce

Preparation Time: 15 minutes

Cooking Time: 15 minutes

Servings: 3

Ingredients:

8 Loin lamb chops

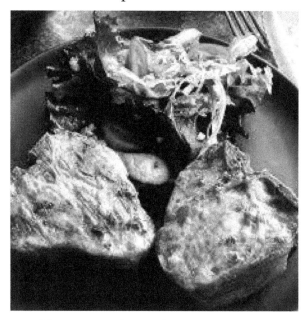

2 Tablespoons olive oil

1 Tablespoon garlic (minced)

1 Tablespoon kosher salt

1 Tablespoon pepper

Horseradish cream sauce

1 Tablespoon Dijon mustard

2 Tablespoons sugar

½ Cup mayonnaise

2 Tablespoon horseradish (prepared)

Directions

The mustard, sugar, mayonnaise and horseradish should be mixed in a bowl and stirred to form a consistent mixture. The mixture should be divided into two parts. The air fryer toaster oven should be preheated at 325 F for 5 min. The lamb chops are placed in the basket and heated for 10 min with intermittent flipping. The cooked lambs are removed from the basket, placed in the bowl containing sauce. The chops are turned on all sides for even coating. The lamb chops are placed in the basket of the air fryer and heated ay 390°F further for 5 min with intermittent flipping. The cooked lamb should be removed from the basket and served hot with horseradish sauce.

Nutrition

Calories: 623 kcal/Cal

Fat: 53 g

Carbs: 4 g

 Protein: 31 g

Lamb Chops in Greek style

Preparation Time: 5 minutes

Cooking Time: 15 minutes

Servings: 4

Ingredients:

8 Loin lamb chops

2 Tablespoons olive oil

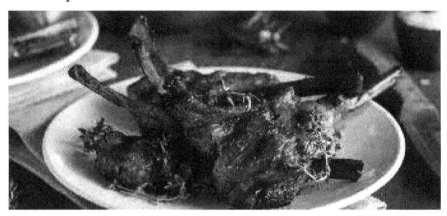

4 Table spoons grainy Mustard

1 Table spoon Greek oregano

¼ Tablespoon pepper

¼ Tablespoon salt

1 Tablespoon thyme

Directions

The mustard, thyme, oregano and olive oil are mixed thoroughly in a bowl. The lamb chops should be rinsed and dried. The prepared mixture is coated on the lamb chops. The air fryer toaster oven should be preheated at 390°F for 5 min. The lambs are placed assembled pan into rack Position and heated for 15 min with intermittent flipping. The cooked lamb should be removed from the basket and served hot.

Nutrition

Calories: 265 kcal/Cal

Fat: 40 g

Carbs: 4 g

Protein: 30 g

Garlic Lemon Shrimp

Preparation Time: 35 minutes

Cooking Time: 10 minutes

Servings: 3

Ingredients:

1 lb. Shrimp, peeled

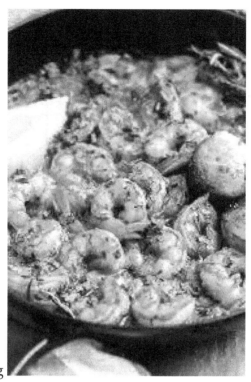

Fish seasoning

2 Tablespoons olive oil

¼ Tablespoon chili flakes

1 Tablespoon garlic (minced)

¼ Tablespoon pepper

¼ Tablespoon salt

1 Lemon (sliced)

Directions

The fish seasoning is mixed thoroughly and placed in a zip lock bag. The shrimp are added to the bag and allowed to marinade for 30 min. The air fryer toaster oven should be preheated at 390°F for 5 min. The shrimp are placed in the assembled pan into rack Position and heated for 8 min with intermittent flipping. The cooked pink shrimp should be removed from the basket and served with lemon.

Nutrition

Calories: 228 kcal/Cal

Fat: 2 g

Carbs: 16 g

Protein: 14.2 g

Chapter 4: Dinner Recipes

Mouthwatering Shredded BBQ Roast

Preparation Time: 10 minutes

Cooking Time: 30 minutes

Servings: 8

Ingredients:

4 lbs. pork roast

1 tsp. garlic powder

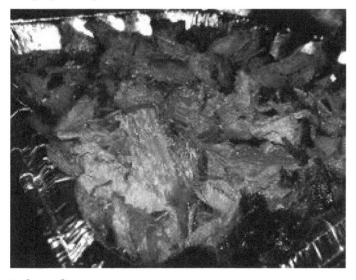

Salt and pepper to taste

1/2 cup water

2 can (11 oz.) of barbecue sauce, keno unsweetened

Directions:

Season the pork with garlic powder, salt and pepper, place in your Instant Pot.

Pour water and lock lid into place; set on the MEAT/STEW, high pressure setting for 30 minutes.

When ready, use Quick Release - turn the valve from sealing to venting to release the pressure.

Remove pork in a bowl, and with two forks shred the meat.

Pour BBQ sauce and stir to combine well.

Serve.

Nutrition:

Calories: 373 kcal/Cal

Carbohydrates: 2.5 g

Proteins: 34 g

Fat: 24 g

Fiber: 3 g

Sour and Spicy Spareribs

Preparation Time: 15 minutes

Cooking Time: 35 minutes

Servings: 10

Ingredients

5 lbs. spare spareribs

Salt and pepper to taste

2 Tbsp. of tallow

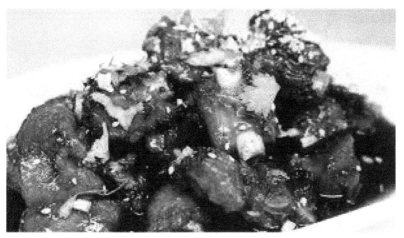

1/2 cup coconut amines (from coconut sap)

1/2 cup vinegar

2 Tbsp. Worcestershire sauce, to taste

1 tsp. chili powder

1 tsp. garlic powder

1 tsp. celery seeds

Directions:

Cut the rack of ribs into equal portions.

Season salt and ground pepper your spareribs from all sides.

Add tallow in your Instant Pot and place spareribs.

In a bowl, combine all remaining ingredients and pour over spareribs.

Lock lid into place and set on the MANUAL setting on HIGH heat for 35 minutes.

When the timer beeps, press "Cancel" and carefully flip the Natural Release for 20 minutes.

Open the lid and transfer ribs on a serving platter.

Serve hot.

Nutrition:

Calories: 598 kcal/Cal

Carbohydrates: 2 g

Proteins: 36 g

Fat: 54 g

Fiber: 0.2 g

Tender Pork Shoulder with Hot Peppers

Preparation Time: 10 minutes

Cooking Time: 30 minutes

Servings: 8

Ingredients:

3 lbs. pork shoulder boneless

Salt and ground black pepper to taste

3 Tbsp. of olive oil

1 large onion, chopped

2 cloves garlic minced

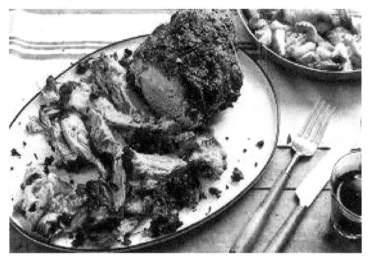

2 - 3 chili peppers, chopped

1 tsp. ground coriander

1 tsp. ground cumin

1 ½ cups of bone broth (preferably homemade)

1/2 cup water

Directions:

Season salt and pepper the pork meat.

Turn on the Instant Pot and press SAUTÉ button. When the word "hot" appears on the display, add the oil and sauté the onions and garlic about 5 minutes.

Add pork and sear for 1 - 2 minutes from all sides; turn off the SAUTÉ button.

Add all remaining ingredients into Instant Pot.

Lock lid into place and set on the MEAT/STEW setting on HIGH heat for 30 minutes.

When the timer beeps, press "Cancel" and carefully flip the Natural Release button for 15 minutes. Serve hot.

Nutrition:

Calories: 389 kcal/Cal

Carbohydrates: 2.5 g

Proteins: 36 g

Fat: 27 g

Fiber: 0.5 g

Braised Sour Pork Filet

Preparation Time: 10 minutes

Cooking Time: 8 hours

Servings: 6

Ingredients:

1/2 tsp. of dry thyme

1/2 tsp. of sage

Salt and ground black pepper to taste

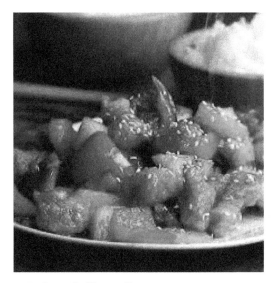

2 Tabs of olive oil

3 lbs. of pork fillet

1/3 cup of shallots (chopped)

3 cloves of garlic (minced)

3/4 cup of bone broth

1/3 cup of apple cider vinegar

Directions:

In a small bowl, combine thyme, sage, salt and black ground pepper.

Rub generously pork from all sides.

Heat the olive oil in a large frying pan, and sear pork for 2 - 3 minutes.

Place pork in your Crock Pot and add shallots and garlic.

Pour broth and apple cider vinegar / juice.

Cover and cook on SLOW for 8 hours or on HIGH for 4-5 hours.

Remove pork on a plate, adjust salt and pepper, slice and serve with cooking juice.

Nutrition:

Calories: 348 kcal/Cal

Carbohydrates: 3 g

Proteins: 51 g

Fat: 12.5 g

Fiber: 0.1 g

Pork with Anise and Cumin Stir-fry

Preparation Time: 5 minutes

Cooking Time: 30 minutes

Servings: 4

Ingredients:

2 Tbsp. lard

2 spring onions finely chopped (only green part)

2 cloves garlic, finely chopped

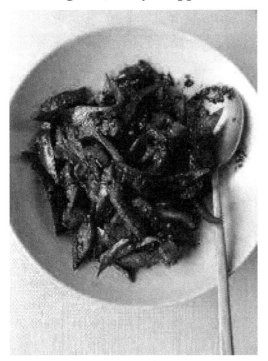

2 lbs. pork loin, boneless, cut into cubes

Sea salt and black ground pepper to taste

1 green bell pepper (cut into thin strips)

1/2 cup water

1/2 tsp. dill seeds

1/2 anise seeds

1/2 tsp. cumin

Directions:

Heat the lard n a large frying pot over medium-high heat.

Sauté the spring onions and garlic with a pinch of salt for 3 - 4 minutes.

Add the pork and simmer for about 5 - 6 minutes.

Add all remaining ingredients and stir well.

Cover and let simmer for 15 - 20 minutes

Taste and adjust seasoning to taste.

Serve!

Nutrition:

Calories: 351 kcal/Cal

Carbohydrates: 3 g

Proteins: 1 g

Fat: 51.5 g

Fiber: 1 g

Baked Meatballs with Goat Cheese

Preparation Time: 15 minutes

Cooking Time: 35 minutes

Servings: 8

Ingredients:

1 Tbsp. of tallow

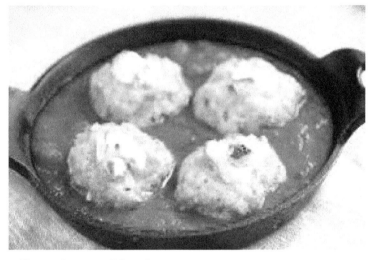

2 lbs. of ground beef

1 organic egg

1 grated onion

1/2 cup of almond milk (unsweetened)

1 cup of red wine

1/2 bunch of chopped parsley

1/2 cup of almond flour

Salt and ground pepper to taste

1/2 Tbsp. of dry oregano

4 oz. of hard goat cheese cut in cubes

Directions:

Preheat oven to 400°F.

Grease a baking pan with tallow.

In a large bowl, combine all ingredients except goat cheese.

Knead the mixture until ingredients are evenly combined.

Make small meatballs and place in a prepared baking dish.

Place one cube of cheese on each meatball.

Bake for 30 - 35 minutes.

Serve hot.

Nutrition:

Calories: 404 kcal/Cal

Carbohydrates: 2.2 g

Proteins: 25.5 g

Fat: 31 g

Fiber: 0.5 g

Parisian Schnitzel

Preparation Time: 15 minutes

Cooking Time: 10 minutes

Servings: 4

Ingredients:

4 veal steaks; thin schnitzel

Salt and ground black pepper

2 Tbsp. of butter

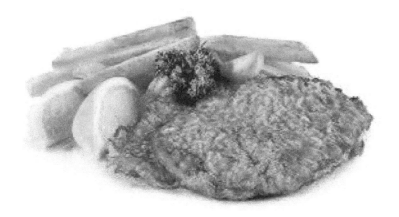

3 eggs from free-range chickens

4 Tbsp. of almond flour

Directions:

Season steaks with the salt and pepper.

Heat butter in a large nonstick frying pan at medium heat.

In a bowl, beat the eggs.

Add almond flour in a bowl.

Roll each steak in almond flour, add then, dip in beaten eggs.

Fry about 3 minutes per side.

Serve right away.

Nutrition:

Calories: 355 kcal/Cal

Carbohydrates: 0.3 g

Proteins: 54 g

Fat: 15 g

Fiber: 0 g

Kato Beef Stroganoff

Preparation Time: 5 minutes

Cooking Time: 30 minutes

Servings: 6

 Ingredients:

2 lbs. of rump or round steak or stewing steak

4 Tbsp. of olive oil

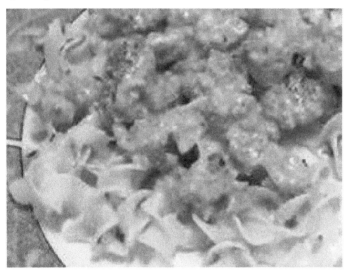

2 green onions, finely chopped

1 grated tomato

2 Tbsp. ketchup (without sugar)

1 cup of button mushrooms

1/2 cup of bone broth

1 cup of sour cream

Salt and black pepper to taste

Directions:

Cut the meat into strips and sauté in large frying skillet.

Add chopped onion and a pinch of salt and cook meat for about 20 minutes at medium temperature.

Add mushrooms and ketchup and stir for 3 - 5 minutes.

Pour the bone broth and sour cream and cook for 3 - 4 minutes.

Remove from the heat, taste and adjust salt and pepper to taste.

Serve hot.

Nutrition:

Calories: 348 kcal/Cal

Carbohydrates: 4.2 g

Proteins: 37 g

Fat: 21 g

Fiber: 1 g

CPSIA information can be obtained
at www.ICGtesting.com
Printed in the USA
BVHW011710160321
602658BV00006B/303

9 781802 229394